# Dr Sebi Cure For Herpes

*37 Alkaline Diet To Cure Herpes Virus Naturally That You Must Know To Get Rid Of Cold Sore And Genital Herpes*

James Andrew Brian

Copyright © 2022 by James Andrew Brian

All rights reserved. No part of this publication may be reproduced, distributed, or transmitted in any form or by any means, including photocopying, recording, or other electronic or mechanical methods, without the prior written permission of the publisher, except in the case of brief quotations embodied in critical reviews and certain other non-commercial uses permitted by copyright law.

# Table of Contents

Dr Sebi Cure For Herpes ................................................. 1

INTRODUCTION .............................................................. 5

CHAPTER 1 ..................................................................... 9

    Genital Herpes ............................................................ 9

CHAPTER 2 ................................................................... 22

    Is The Dr. Sebi Diet A Good Idea? ............................ 22

CHAPTER 3 ................................................................... 39

    37 Home Remedies for Herpes Simplex Virus 1 and Virus 2 ........................................................................ 39

CHAPTER 4 ................................................................... 57

    Foods to Avoid When You Have a Cold Sore ........... 57

CHAPTER 5 ................................................................... 60

    How do I obtain herpes treatment? ........................... 60

CHAPTER 6 ................................................................... 80

    What causes female vaginal sores? ........................... 80

CHAPTER 7 ................................................................... 87

    How do you deal with herpes on a long-term basis? . 87

CHAPTER 8 ................................................................... 94

    At-home herpes treatment ......................................... 94

Acknowledgments ................................ 111

# INTRODUCTION

More than 100 million people live with the chronic and frequently painful disease, according to the World Health Organization.

Dr. Sebi has been in the world longer than the average person and has seen more than they can imagine, so you should pay heed when he says that herpes can be healed with just a few herbs.

Herpes is a disease that we've all heard of but are embarrassed to confess. Therefore, most of us have no idea how it works or how to treat it.

We put this book together with the assistance of Dr. Sebi (diet guidelines), who has been utilizing natural cures for herpes and other sexually transmitted illnesses for years and is now ready to share what he has discovered with the rest of the world. Dr. Sebi is a big fan of natural medicine. He has spent his whole career studying plants and how they affect the body.

What Is Herpes and How Does It Affect You? Herpes is one of the most common STDs and is caused by the herpes simplex virus (HSV). Oral sex, anal intercourse, vaginal sex, and even kissing are all ways to contract it. The virus can also be passed from mother to child during pregnancy or childbirth in some situations. In most circumstances, the person who has been infected with herpes will have no symptoms at first. If the virus spreads to the genitals, however, it can cause skin sores or blisters, which can lead to fever, headaches, sore throats, and swollen glands. Only about 20 herpes viruses are known to infect people, despite the fact that there are over 100 varieties of herpes viruses. HSV-1 and HSV-2 are the two most frequent kinds among them.

While nearly everyone has been infected with HSV-1 at some point in their lives, most individuals will only be infected with HSV-2 once. It is conceivable for a person to contract herpes twice, but this is extremely rare. How Is Herpes Detected? Taking a blood sample to test for the presence of antibodies is the first step in diagnosing herpes. When the immune system senses an infection, antibodies are created. Herpes can be spread without causing any symptoms since it is transmitted through sexual contact. As a result, even if there are no obvious symptoms, the existence of antibodies might establish the diagnosis. If a blood test reveals that the patient lacks antibodies, a doctor can examine other samples to see if a specific virus is present. What Is Herpes and How Does It Work? The virus enters our bodies through our genitals or mouth when we have sex with someone. The virus then goes through our circulation to nerve cells in our genitals and brain, where it remains dormant. This dormant virus remains in nerve cells and produces the glycoprotein C protein. The virus then hides in this protein, allowing it to avoid being detected by the immune system. The virus can still reproduce at this time, but it can't because the immune system has discovered it. The immune system continues to battle the virus by producing antibodies that bind to it and eliminate it. The virus, on the other hand, always returns and strives to replicate itself. This cycle repeats until the virus's immune system can no longer keep up with it. This is why herpes can be so difficult to eradicate. Is There a Herpes Cure? Herpes is usually not lethal, but it can bring a slew of issues. As a result, many people opt to treat their herpes infection using natural remedies.

Herpes is a virus that can be treated with herbal remedies. I also use the same method to treat herpes. Numerous studies have confirmed this.

It also has no negative side effects. It's a safe and effective technique to treat and prevent herpes. In this book, I'm going to tell you everything you need to know about this remedy.

# CHAPTER 1

## Genital Herpes

Herpes simplex virus type 1 (HSV-1) or type 2 causes genital herpes, a sexually transmitted illness (STD) (HSV-2).

### *What is the prevalence of genital herpes?*

Infection with genital herpes is very common in the United States. In a single year, the CDC projected that 572,000 new genital herpes infections occurred in the United States. In the United States, HSV-2 infection affects 11.9 percent of people aged 14 to 49 (12.1 percent when adjusted for age). However, because HSV-1 is causing an increasing number of genital herpes infections, the prevalence of genital herpes infections has increased. Because the prevalence of oral HSV-1 infection has decreased in recent decades, people may be more susceptible to getting a genital herpes infection from

HSV-1.

HSV-2 infection is more common in women than in men; among 14–49-year-olds, the percentages of those affected in 2015–2016 were 15.9% versus 8.2%, respectively. This could be because genital infections are more easily transmitted from men to women during penile-vaginal sex than from women to men. Non-Hispanic blacks (34.6 percent) are more likely than non-Hispanic whites (8.1 percent) to be infected with HSV-2. According to a prior study, these differences exist even among those who have had the same number of lifetime sexual partners. In the United States, an estimated 87.4% of 14–49-year-olds infected with HSV-2 have never had a clinical diagnosis.

### *How can a person contract genital herpes?*

Contact with HSV in herpes lesions, mucosal surfaces, vaginal secretions, or oral secretions transmits infections. HSV-1 and HSV-2 can be shed from healthy oral and vaginal mucosa and skin. In most cases, HSV-2 infection can only be contracted through vaginal contact with someone who has genital HSV-2 infection. Receiving oral sex from someone who has an oral HSV-1 infection, on the other hand, can result in a genital HSV-1 infection. Contact with an infected partner who does not have obvious lesions and may not be aware that he or she is afflicted is the most prevalent method of transmission. Genital HSV shedding occurred on 10.2 percent of days in people with asymptomatic HSV-2 infections, compared to 20.1 percent of days in people with symptomatic infections.

## *What are some of the signs and symptoms of genital herpes?*

The majority of HSV patients are asymptomatic or have extremely mild symptoms that go unreported or are misdiagnosed as another skin condition. When symptoms do occur, one or more vesicles, or small blisters, appear on or around the genitals, rectum, or mouth. After exposure, the typical incubation period for an initial herpes infection is 4 days (range: 2 to 12). After the herpes infection, the vesicles rupture and leave painful ulcers that might take two to four weeks to heal. First herpes "outbreak" or "episode" is defined as the occurrence of these symptoms. The first and recurrent (i.e., subsequent) outbreaks of genital herpes have different clinical symptoms. The first herpes outbreak is generally accompanied by a longer duration of herpetic lesions, higher viral shedding (which makes HSV transmission more likely), and systemic symptoms such as fever, body aches, swollen lymph nodes, or headache. Many patients who detect recurrences have prodromal symptoms such as localized genital pain or tingling or shooting sensations in the legs, hips, or buttocks, which occur hours to days before the development of herpetic lesions. Recurrent episodes of genital herpes usually last less time and are less severe than the initial epidemic. According to long-term studies, the number of symptomatic recurrent outbreaks may decrease over time.

When it comes to genital HSV-1 infection, recurrences and subclinical shedding are much less common than when it comes to genital HSV-2 infection.

## *Genital Herpes Complications*

In people with weakened immune systems, such as HIV-positive people, genital herpes can produce painful genital ulcers that can last for months. HSV-1 and HSV-2 can both induce aseptic meningitis, which is a rare but deadly consequence (inflammation of the linings of the brain). During the course of infection, extragenital lesions (e.g., buttocks, groin, thigh, finger, or eye) may develop. Some people with genital herpes worry about how it will affect their overall health, sexual life, and relationships. A herpes diagnosis can also cause significant embarrassment, shame, and stigma, all of which can negatively impact a patient's relationships. Clinicians can alleviate these fears by reassuring patients that, while herpes is incurable, it is a treatable condition.

Giving information, providing support resources, and assisting in the definition of treatment and preventative alternatives are three key measures that clinicians can take for their newly diagnosed patients. Patients can be advised that disclosing their illness to sexual partners, avoiding sex during a recurrent outbreak, using a suppressive antiviral medication, and using condoms consistently will minimize, but not eliminate, the risk of genital herpes transmission. Because a diagnosis of genital herpes might alter how people think about their current or future sexual relationships, it's critical for patients to know how to communicate about STDs with their partners.

***Is there a connection between genital herpes and HIV?***
Herpes causes genital ulcerative illness, which makes it easier to spread and acquire HIV infection through sexual contact. Individuals with genital herpes infection have a 2-to-4-fold increased risk of contracting HIV if they are

genitally exposed to HIV. 13–15 Ulcers or breaks in the skin or mucous membranes (mouth, vaginal, and rectum) caused by a herpes infection can damage the skin's and mucous membranes' normal protection against infections, including HIV. In addition, genital herpes increases the number of CD4 cells in the genital mucosa, which are the cells that HIV can get into. Local activation of HIV replication at the site of genital herpes infection can enhance the risk of HIV transmission during contact with an HIV-uninfected sex partner's mouth, vagina, or rectum in people who have both HIV and genital herpes.

## *What are the effects of genital herpes on a pregnant mother and her baby?*

Neonatal herpes is one of the most dangerous genital herpes complications. Healthcare providers should inquire about genital herpes in all pregnant women. Herpes infections can be spread from mother to child during pregnancy or childbirth, or babies might contact them shortly after birth, leading to a potentially fatal neonatal herpes infection. Compared to infants delivered to mothers who have acquired genital herpes close to the time of birth and are shedding the virus at delivery, they are at a substantially higher risk of getting neonatal herpes. 16, 18-20 As a result, it is critical for women to avoid getting herpes during pregnancy. Women should be told not to have sex with partners who have or are suspected of having genital herpes during the third trimester.

While antiviral medicine may be given to women with genital herpes late in pregnancy through delivery to lower the chance of a recurring outbreak, third-trimester antiviral prophylaxis has not been shown to lessen the risk of herpes transmission to the newborn.

Pregnant women should not be screened for HSV regularly. At the commencement of labor, however, all women should be thoroughly examined and questioned to rule out the presence of prodromal symptoms or herpetic lesions. If herpes symptoms are present, a cesarean delivery should be performed to stop HSV from spreading to the newborn.

### *How do you know if you have genital herpes?*

The HSV nucleic acid amplification tests (NAAT) are the most sensitive and specific herpes testing available. In some cases, however, viral culture is the only test available. Viral culture has low sensitivity, especially in people with recurrent or healing lesions. Because viral shedding is intermittent, it is possible to have a genital herpes infection even if NAAT or culture did not reveal it. When a person has recurring symptoms or a lesion without a confirmatory NAAT or culture result or has a partner with genital herpes, type-specific virologic tests can be performed to diagnose genital herpes. In healthcare settings serving patients with or at risk for sexually transmitted infections, both virologic assays and type-specific serologic tests should be accessible.

Because commercially available type-specific serologic tests have limitations, particularly with low index value results, a confirmatory test (Biokit or Western Blot) using a different method should be done before test interpretation. Patients should be advised about the limitations of available testing before serologic testing if confirmatory tests are unavailable. False-positive results do happen, and healthcare providers should be aware of this. Having a blood test done within 12 weeks of a suspected recent acquisition may lead to false-negative results.

Serologic testing for HSV-1 does not distinguish between oral and genital infections, hence it is rarely used to diagnose genital HSV-1 infection. Virologic tests from lesions confirm the diagnosis of genital HSV-1 infection. Due to the limits of type-specific serologic testing, the CDC does not recommend screening for HSV-1 or HSV-2 in the general population. There are several instances in which type-specific serologic HSV tests may be beneficial:

Patients presenting with unusual or recurring genital symptoms and a negative HSV NAAT or culture;

Patients who have a clinical diagnosis of genital herpes but no laboratory confirmation; and patients who have a clinical diagnosis of genital herpes but no laboratory confirmation.

***Patients who have a genital herpes-infected companion***

Patients with HIV and those at increased risk of infection (e.g., those presenting for an STI examination, especially those with many sex partners), may need to be examined for a history of genital herpes symptoms, followed by serology testing in those with genital symptoms.

***Is there a way to get rid of herpes?***

Herpes has no treatment. Antiviral medications, on the other hand, can help to prevent or shorten outbreaks while they are being taken. Furthermore, daily suppressive therapy (i.e., taking antiviral medicine on a daily basis) for herpes can lower the risk of transmission to partners. There is no commercially available vaccination that protects against genital herpes infection at this time. Candidate vaccines are currently being tested in clinical trials.

## *What can be done to prevent herpes?*

Because herpes virus shedding can occur in locations not covered by a condom, proper and consistent use of latex condoms can minimize the risk of transmitting or contracting genital herpes. Abstinence from sexual contact or being in a long-term mutually monogamous relationship with a partner who has been tested for STDs and is known to be uninfected are the best ways to avoid transmission of STDs, including genital herpes.

When herpes lesions or other viral symptoms are present, people with herpes should avoid sexual activity with their partners. It's vital to remember that even if a person is symptom-free, he or she can still infect sex partners. Infected persons' sex partners should be informed that they may become infected and should use condoms to limit the risk of infection. Sex partners might have HSV testing done to see if they are infected.

Daily therapy with valacyclovir reduces the rate of HSV-2 transmission in discordant, heterosexual couples where the source spouse has a history of genital HSV-2 infection. In addition to using condoms and not having sex during recurrences, such couples should be told to take suppressive antiviral medication as part of a plan to stop the spread of the virus. It is vital to provide counseling to people who have genital herpes and their sex partners. It can assist patients in coping with the infection and prevent it from spreading further into the community.

# CHAPTER 2

## Is The Dr. Sebi Diet A Good Idea?

Dr. Sebi believed acidity and mucus caused disease. Sebi believed certain foods could be eaten, and others avoided to detoxify the body and achieve an alkaline state, lowering the disease's risk. Official sources have not approved the Dr. Sebi diet, and there is no scientific evidence to support its use in treating or preventing medical conditions. While plant-based diets may be beneficial for some, the Dr. Sebi diet may lack key nutrients that will keep your body healthy.

### Who's Dr. Sebi?

Alfredo Bowman, also known as Dr. Sebi, was a self-described healer and herbalist. He was not a doctor, nor did he have a PhD and was self-educated.

An obituary highlights his controversial claims about

curing AIDS or leukemia. These and other claims led to a 1993 lawsuit in which the court ordered Dr. Sebi's organization to cease making such claims. According to reports, Dr. Sebi died in police custody in 2016.

## What's the Dr. Sebi Diet?

Dr. Sebi thought that the Western approach to diseases was ineffective. Sebi believed that acidity and mucus, rather than bacteria and viruses, caused disease.

The diet's main idea is that disease cannot survive in acidic environments. To prevent or eliminate disease, the diet aims to create an alkaline body.

The diet's official website sells botanical remedies that it claims will detoxify the body. These remedies, called African Bio-mineral balance supplements, retail for $1500 per pack.

It links to no research supporting its claims of health benefits. The site does not mention that the Food and Drug Administration (FDA) statements have been evaluated. The site creators acknowledge they are not doctors and that the site does not replace medical advice.

## How to Follow the Diet

Dr. Sebi's nutritional guide includes several rules, such as:

- Only eat the foods in this guide.
- You need to drink 1 gallon of spring water daily.
- Eating animal products, hybrid food, and alcohol highly need to be reduced.
- You need to avoid using a microwave as it will "kill" your food.
- Canned and seedless fruits should be avoided.

Dr. Sebi's diet includes eating:

- Vegetables such as avocado, bell peppers, and wild arugula
- Fruits such as apples, bananas, and dates.
- You can find grains such as rye, wild Rice.

- Oils such as avocado, hemp seed, and coconut oil, but the diet recommends against the latter two for cooking.

- Nuts and seeds, such as hemp, raw sesame seed, tahini butter, and walnuts

- Herbal teas include chamomile, ginger, and fennel.

- Date sugar and agave syrup

- spices, including cayenne and powdered seaweed

## What are the advantages?

Any scientific evidence does not support the Dr. Sebi diet. Research shows that a plant-based diet is good for your health. We will discuss the risks in the next section. There are some health benefits to plant-based diets, such as:

***Weight loss:*** -- 2015 Study Participants lost up to 7.5% more weight on a vegan diet than those following stricter diets. Participants lost as much as 7.5%. Bodyweight after six months on a vegan diet.

***Controlling your appetite:--*** 2016 Study Young male participants discovered that eating a plant-based meal with beans and peas made them feel fuller than when they ate meat.

Modifying the microbiome term "microbiome" refers collectively to the microorganisms found in the gut. A 2019 study found that a plant-based diet can alter the microbiome positively, leading to a lower risk of developing diseases. This will need to be confirmed, however.

***Lower risk of developing a disease:--*** It was concluded that a plant-based diet could reduce the risk of developing AIDS. Coronary heart disease by 40%, the risk of developing metabolic syndrome, type 2 Diabetes.

Eating whole foods is greatly advised by Dr. Sebi's Diet rather than consuming processed foods. It was discovered from a study in 2017 that reducing the intake of processed food would improve the nutritional quality of the general diet in the United States.

## The Downsides to the Dr. Sebi diet

Dr. Sebi's diet has a significant drawback. It restricts many food groups, including animal products, wheat and beans, and many other vegetables and fruits.

It's so strict that it allows only certain types of fruit. You can eat plum or cherry tomatoes, but not other types like beefsteak and Roma tomatoes.

A restrictive diet can also be unpleasant and cause a bad relationship with food. This is especially true if you don't like foods not listed in the nutrition guide.

This diet encourages unhealthy eating habits, such as taking supplements to gain fullness. This claim, which claims that supplements are not a significant source of calories, encourages unhealthy eating habits—deficient in protein and other vital nutrients.

***These foods can be a great source of nutrition.***

None of these foods is a good source of protein. This essential nutrient helps with skin structure, muscle growth, and hormone production.

Brazil nuts, sesame, and hemp seeds are all allowed, but they aren't excellent protein sources. A 1/4 cup (25g) of walnuts or 3 tbsp (30g) of hemp seeds will provide four and 9grams, respectively.

You would need to consume large amounts of these foods to meet your daily protein requirements. Although foods from this diet contain high amounts of certain nutrients such as beta carotene and potassium and vitamins C, E, and vitamins, they are low in vitamins D, iron, calcium, and vitamin D and B12. These nutrients are essential for people who eat a strictly plant-based diet.

According to Dr. Sebi, certain ingredients in his supplements are proprietary. This is concerning as it makes it hard to determine if you will meet your daily nutritional needs.

It is not based on science. Dr. Sebi's diet plan is criticized for not having enough scientific evidence. He claims that your body's acid production is controlled by the foods and supplements you eat. The human body regulates acid-base balance to maintain blood pH levels between 7.36 & 7.44. This naturally makes your body slightly alkaline.

Rare cases such as diabetes ketoacidosis, where blood pH may be out of range, can lead to death. This can lead to death if not treated immediately.

Research has also shown that while your diet can temporarily and slightly alter your urine pH, it will not affect your blood pH. Following Dr. Sebi's diet won't make your body less alkaline.

### Foods to Eat

Dr. Sebi's nutrition guidance details the foods that are allowed in his diet.

- Fruits: apples, cantaloupe, currants, dates, figs, elderberries, papayas, berries, peaches, soft jelly coconuts, pears, plums, seeded vital limes, mangoes, prickly pears, seeded melons, Latin or West Indies soursop, tamarind.

- Vegetable bell peppers and cactus flowers, chickpeas. Avocado.

- Grains:- Fonio (amaranth), Khorasan wheat, Kamut, rye, wild Rice, spelled and teff.

- Seeds and Nuts:- Brazil nuts. Hemp seeds. Raw sesame seeds. Raw tahini butter. Walnuts.

- Oils:- Avocado, coconut oil (uncooked), grapeseed, hempseed, olive oil, sesame oil

- Herbal teas:- Elderberry, chamomile, fennel, tila, burdock, ginger, raspberry

- Spices:- Oregano and basil, cloves bay leaf, sweet basil. Achiote. Habanero. Tarragon. Onion powder. Sage. Pure sea salt. Thyme. Pure agave syrup. date sugar

- You can also drink water, in addition to tea.

- You can also eat allowed grains such as pasta,

cereals, bread, and flour. All food that is leavened or baked with yeast and baking powder is prohibited.

**Foods to Avoid**

All foods not listed in the Dr. Sebi nutrition guides are prohibited, including:

- Cans of fruit and vegetables
- Seedless fruit
- Eggs
- Dairy
- Fish
- Red meat
- Poultry
- Soy products

Take-out and restaurant food are all acceptable options

for processed food

- Fortified foods

- Wheat

- Sugar (aside from date sugar and Agave syrup)

- Alcohol

- Foods or yeast-based yeast products

- Baking powder can be used to make delicious foods

- The diet bans many fruits, vegetables, grains, nuts, seeds, and legumes.

- Only the foods in the guide can be eaten.

### Sample menu

Below is a sample menu for Dr. Sebi's three-day diet.

### Day 1

***Breakfast:*** 2 Banana-spelt pancakes with Agave syrup

Snack1 Cup (240ml) green juice smoothie made from

cucumbers, kale, and apples

*Lunch:* kale salad with tomatoes, onions, and dandelion greens. Also, chickpeas with olive oils and basil dressing.

*Dinner:* Vegetable and Wild-rice Stir-Fry

## Day 2

*Breakfast:* shake with water, hemp seed, bananas, and strawberries

*Snack:-* blueberry muffins made from blueberries, pure coconut milk, agave syrup, and oil.

*Lunch:-* a homemade pie made with a spelled flour crust, Brazil-nut Cheese, and your choice of vegetables

Snacktahini butter on Rye Bread with Sliced Red Peppers

*Dinner:-* Chickpea Burger with Tomato, Onion, and Kale on spelled flour flatbread

## Day 3

*Breakfast:-* Cooked Quinoa with pure coconut milk, peaches, and agave syrup, Snack chamomile, seeded grapes, and sesame seeds

*Lunch:-* Spaghetti salad with chopped vegetables, olive

oil, and key lime dressing

***Snack:-*** A smoothie made with mango and bananas, pure coconut milk, and pure coconut oil

***Dinner:-*** Hearty vegetable soup with mushrooms, red peppers, and zucchini.

## Is it safe to use?

Dr. Sebi's diet is strict and may not contain enough nutrients. This is not something that Dr Sebi acknowledges.

A person who adopts this diet may find it beneficial to consult a healthcare professional to see if they need additional supplements.

## Vitamin B-12

Following the Dr. Sebi diet may result in a vitamin B-12 deficiency. Supplements and fortified food may help to prevent this. Vitamin B-12 is an essential nutrient necessary for nerve and blood cells' health and making DNA. People who eat vegan or vegetarian diets and older adults are at greater risk for B-12 deficiencies. People who don't eat animal products should take B-12 supplements.

B-12 deficiencies can lead to tiredness, depression, and tingling in your hands and feet. Pernicious anemia is another possibility. This prevents the body from making enough healthy red blood cells.

**Protein**

Protein helps support the brain's health, muscles, bones, hormones, and DNA in the diet.

According to current guidelines, females over 19 should have a daily protein intake of 46grams(g), while males of the same age should consume 56g.

Protein is found in some foods that are part of the Dr. Sebi Diet. 100g of hulled hemp seed contains 31.56g of protein. The exact amount of walnuts has of 16.67g of protein. For comparison, 100 g of oven-roasted chicken breast contains 16.79 g of the nutrient.

However, Dr. Sebi's diet restricts other plant protein sources, such as beans, lentils, and soy. To meet their daily protein needs, a person would have to consume many of the allowed protein sources.

Research suggests that it is vital to eat a wide variety of plant foods to absorb enough amino acids, building blocks of protein. One thing I want you to know is that Dr. Sebi's diet can be tasking to follow.

**The Immune System**

Omega-3s is the vital plant source when it comes to Dr. Sebi's Diet, such as hemp seeds and walnuts. This helps the body to easily absorbs these acids from animal sources. According to a 2019 study, vegans are less likely to consume the two essential omega-3 fatty acids unless they supplement. An omega-3 supplement may be beneficial for anyone following the Dr. Sebi Diet.

**Recipes**

Many of Dr. Sebi's recipes contain unusual ingredients

and his patent-pending botanical supplements. A person may not strictly follow the diet but adapt specific recipes to create healthy, plant-based meals.

*Dr. Sebi's "veggie-ful" smoothie.* You can leave out the date sugar as the drink might be sweet enough without it.

*Zucchini bread pancakes.* Sugar can be replaced with maple syrup or coconut sugar.

*Veggie fajitas tacos.* These types of tortillas may be more appealing to people who eat wheat or corn.

The Dr. Sebi diet has not been supported by scientific research. It may offer some of the same benefits as other plant-based diets.

Health benefits could be achieved by eating more whole fruits, vegetables, and legumes. If weight loss is your goal, it could be a great way to eat more whole fruits and vegetables.

However, Dr. Sebi's restrictions could present risks. It is important to ensure that your body gets enough nutrients, including vitamin B-12, through supplementation if needed. Some people are more vulnerable to Dr. Sebi's risks. These include adolescents, breastfeeding women, and older adults.

Proponents of the diet recommend expensive products, but no scientific evidence supports their usage. You could eat more plants and supplement with nutrients to be more healthy. Before you try a new diet, it is good to do some research and talk to a professional.

# CHAPTER 3

## 37 Home Remedies for Herpes Simplex Virus 1 and Virus 2

Nutritional science appears to produce a steady stream of studies indicating the health benefits of eating a variety of vegetables, particularly those in the brassica family, such as broccoli, cabbage, and cauliflower. According to studies, indole-3-carbinol, a component of brassica vegetables, has the potential to protect against a variety of cancers, including breast and prostate cancers. In a recent study, Indole-3-carbinol was also discovered to have the ability to block the herpes simplex virus, which causes cold sores.

The herpes virus remains dormant in the body once it has been contracted, where it is typically kept under control by the immune system. There are some times when the herpes virus can come back and cause a cold sore to appear on the surface of the skin. These are times when we are tired and our immune systems are weak. The amino acid arginine, which is abundant in chocolate and peanuts, aids and abets the replication of the herpes virus. In the long run, chocolate peanuts appear to be one meal to avoid if you want to prevent cold sores. While arginine aggravates the herpes simplex virus, lysine, on the other hand, has the opposite effect. Lysine, like indole-3-carbinol, suppresses the herpes virus by thwarting its ability to proliferate in the body. While consuming foods high in lysine (such as bananas) has the potential to help prevent cold sores in theory, in practice, a more aggressive strategy works better. Taking 1,000 mg of lysine in the form of a supplement every day can help to reduce the incidence of cold-sore outbreaks. If signs of an eruption threaten, such as pain, numbness, or tingling in the skin, a higher dose is usually required. At the first hint of problems, taking 1 gram of lysine three times a day for a few days can typically stop an assault in its tracks. It doesn't matter whether you already have a cold sore or not. Lysine supplements have been shown to help lessen the severity of cold sores and speed up their healing.

Vitamin C, which has both immune-stimulating and antiviral characteristics, is another natural substance that works well with lysine. A daily dose of 1 g of vitamin C is effective as a preventative, but if a full-blown cold sore or approaching signs are present, a three-times-a-day dose is recommended.

Cold sore sufferers may benefit from lotions or ointments containing aloe vera or propolis for topical relief (a natural antimicrobial agent extracted from beehives). Both of these compounds have been reported to help relieve the pain and speed up the healing of cold sores.

According to experience, natural therapies provide a lot of lip service for cold-sore sufferers. These tried-and-true home remedies may help relieve swelling, itching, and stinging caused by outbreaks. In your kitchen cabinet or medicine chest, you most likely already have everything you need for these treatments.

## Compresses That Are Warm

A preliminary study suggests that applying heat as soon as you notice a pain developing may be beneficial. Heat may assist in reducing discomfort and swelling if a sore has already formed. Fill a sock halfway with rice and microwave for slightly under a minute to generate a dry heated compress.

### *Apply a cool compress.*

A cold compress can also be used to relieve swelling. Apply ice to the affected area with an ice pack or a clean, soft washcloth loaded with ice. Repeat every 4 hours as needed. Always avoid putting ice directly on the skin.

### *A Baking Soda Paste*

Applying a baking soda paste to lesions can help them dry out and decrease irritation. To do this, dip a damp cotton ball or Q-tip into a small amount of pure baking soda and dab it on the sore.

### *Paste made from cornstarch*

Corn starch paste can also be used to reduce itching and dry out sores. A damp cotton ball or Q-tip can be used to apply a small amount of cornstarch to the area that needs help.

### *Garlic that is applied topically*

According to an older study, garlic may have antiviral capabilities against both herpes types. To dilute, crush a fresh garlic clove and blend it with olive oil. This mixture can be applied to a sore up to three times per day.

### *Apple cider vinegar is used topically (ACV).*

The anti-inflammatory and antiviral effects of ACV are well-known. Mix one part ACV with three parts warm water and apply it to the affected region to get some of these advantages.

### **Changes in diet**

Eating the right foods and avoiding certain things can help your body fight off the herpes virus. According to anecdotal data, changing your diet may help reduce outbreaks.

### *Vegetables high in antioxidants*

Antioxidant-rich foods can help to enhance your immune system and reduce inflammation. Antioxidants that bind free radicals are abundant in cauliflower, spinach, kale, and tomatoes. They also have a higher lysine to arginine ratio, which is helpful for herpes suppression.

### *Omega-3 fatty acids are essential fatty acids.*

Chronic inflammatory disorders of the immune system can be managed by omega-3-chain fatty acids. These fatty acids are abundant in salmon, mackerel, flaxseed, and chia seeds.

### *Protein*

Protein consumption is essential for the body's immune response to the herpes virus and other infections. Eating a high-protein, low-saturated-fat diet that includes almonds, eggs, and oats

### *Vitamin C is a powerful antioxidant.*

According to research, Vitamin C has been shown to effectively hasten the healing of herpes outbreaks. It may also aid in the lengthening of the interval between outbreaks.

Vitamin C is abundant in colorful fruits and vegetables such as bell peppers, oranges, and strawberries. As with mangoes and papayas, these fruits are also high in lysine, but they don't add a lot to your food.

### *Zinc*

Zinc therapy may help you have fewer herpes outbreaks while also extending the period between them. Wheat germ, chickpeas, lamb, and pork can help you get more zinc in your diet.

### *B-complex vitamins*

B vitamins can help your body adapt to the herpes virus by boosting your immune system. Green beans, eggs, spinach, and broccoli are all good sources of vitamin B.

### *Acid should be avoided.*

Cold sores can be broken open by acidic foods before they heal. Acidic foods include fruit juice, beer, sodas, and processed foods. Instead of these foods, opt for water or effervescent seltzer.

### *L-arginine should be avoided.*

When possible, stay away from foods that are high in arginine. This amino acid is very abundant in chocolate, and some individuals believe it can cause herpes symptoms. Instead, opt for a vitamin-dense choice like dried mango or apricots to satisfy your sweet tooth.

***Sugar should not be introduced into your diet.***

Added sugars are converted to acids in your body. For desserts, avoid meals with added sugar and opt for naturally sweet delights like bananas and oranges.

***Processed or preservative-laden foods should be avoided.***

Synthetic preservatives in processed foods may contribute to oxidative stress. Keeping oxidative stress levels low during outbreaks may aid in healing. Remove highly processed foods from your diet, such as frozen dinners, refined grain goods, and candy.

***Avoid consuming alcoholic beverages.***

In your body, alcohol degrades to the same level as sugar. Sugar consumption has been linked to a reduction in white blood cells, which can make outbreaks more likely. If you must drink alcohol, do it in moderation and select a less acidic beverage, such as wine.

## Supplements

Supplements can help by boosting your immune system and keeping your skin from getting worse.

It's worth noting, though, that supplements are not regulated by the FDA in the same way that medicines are. Before using any supplement, you should always consult with a healthcare practitioner. Some supplements may interfere with prescription and over-the-counter drugs.

### *Zinc*

Taking zinc may help you have fewer herpes outbreaks each year. A daily dose of 30 milligrams (mg) may be enough to fight off a herpes outbreak.

### *B-complex vitamins*

All of the B-class vitamins are found in vitamin B complex tablets. These vitamins help you feel more energized, improve your metabolism, and promote healthy cell growth. When the virus is attacking the body during an outbreak, these functions are very important.

Each B vitamin in a B-complex supplement has a different amount in each supplement.

### *Lysine*

Lysine is an amino acid that helps your body digest food and develop healthy cells. Lysine's ability to prevent herpes simplex outbreaks is still being studied. According to some findings, a daily lysine intake of 500 mg to 3,000 mg may be useful.

### *Probiotics*

Certain probiotic strains have been proven to aid in the body's immunological response against herpes infections. Taking probiotics can help your immune system in a variety of ways. The first step is to consume yogurt. Lactobacillus rhamnosus strains in probiotic supplements have been shown to increase immunological function.

### *Herbs, oils, and other topical remedies*

Certain topicals, when used correctly, can assist in expediting healing, alleviating itching, and numbing discomfort.

If you don't dilute many topical chemicals, such as essential oils, they might burn through your skin barrier. Carrier oils, like jojoba and coconut oil, are essential for securely applying for topical medicines. Unless it says otherwise, all of the topicals on this page should be used with a carrier oil. Before running a full application, you should also run a patch test. This is the only method to be sure you're not putting something irritating on a sensitive spot.

Follow these steps to perform a quick patch test:

- Apply the cream on the inside of your forearm.
- Wait at least 24 hours.
- If you get itchy, inflamed, or have other problems with the product, wash the area well and stop using it.
- If you don't have any bad reactions in the first 24 hours, you should be able to apply somewhere else.

Look for topicals that don't require the addition of a carrier oil, such as:

- Aloe vera gel
- Honey made from manuka trees
- An extract of licorice
- An extract of echinacea

For the following topicals, purchase a carrier oil:

- A blend of essential oils (tea tree, chamomile, ginger, thyme, eucalyptus)
- Hazel, which
- An extract of lemon balm
- extract of neem

### *Aloe vera gel is a type of aloe vera that*

Aloe vera has been shown to have wound-healing effects. These characteristics could help to treat and calm herpes lesions. Aloe vera gel that has not been diluted can be applied straight to practically any part of the body.

### *Tea tree oil is a natural antiseptic.*

Tea tree oil contains an antiviral component that has been

demonstrated to aid in the treatment of herpes. Before using tea tree oil on a cold sore or genital herpes, dilute it with a carrier oil.

### Hazel is a type of witchcraft.

The antiviral effects of witch hazel are significant. Some people find that pure witch hazel does not irritate them, while others feel that it stings them. If you have sensitive skin, you should use a diluted solution.

### Manuka honey is a type of honey that comes from New Zealand.

An older study suggests that manuka honey applied topically may be as effective as acyclovir in treating HSV-1 and HSV-2. Manuka honey does not need to be diluted before use.

### Milk from a goat

Herpes simplex can be treated using goat milk, which contains an antiviral ingredient. You can use goat milk straight from the animal without diluting it.

### Chamomile essential oil

According to certain studies, chamomile essential oil has anti-viral and anti-soothing effects that could aid in the treatment of HSV-2. It must be mixed with a carrier oil before use.

### *Ginger essential oil*

On contact, ginger essential oil has the ability to kill the herpes virus. It must be mixed with a carrier oil before use.

### *Thyme essential oil*

Thyme essential oil may also help to combat the herpes virus. It must be mixed with a carrier oil before use.

### *Sage oil from Greece*

The herpes virus may also be fought with Greek sage oil. It must be mixed with a carrier oil before use.

### *Eucalyptus essential oil*

Eucalyptus oil has the potential to be a powerful antiviral in the fight against herpes. It also soothes and aids in the healing process. It must be mixed with a carrier oil before use.

### Oregano oil from Mexico

Carvacrol, a potent antiviral component, is found in Mexican oregano oil. It must be mixed with a carrier oil before use.

### Extract of lemon balm

Lemon balm extract essential oil may help to prevent breakouts and transmission. It must be mixed with a carrier oil before use.

### Extracts of sage and rhubarb combined

According to older research, a topical sage-rhubarb preparation may be as efficient as acyclovir in treating HSV-1 symptoms. A carrier oil must be used to dilute this mixture.

### Licorice extract

The key component in licorice root contains antiviral and anti-inflammatory activities. Because of these qualities, licorice extract appears to be a viable treatment for outbreaks. Licorice can be applied straight without diluting.

### *Extract of Echinacea*

Echinacea extract could be a good antiviral for both types of herpes simplex. It's also an anti-inflammatory, so it might help with current outbreaks. Echinacea extract can be used straight without dilution.

### *Extract of neem*

Neem extract may offer anti-herpes properties as well. Neem extract, in its purest form, is quite strong and may cause skin irritation. It must be mixed with a carrier oil before use.

### Do's and don'ts in general

Here are some broad guidelines for dealing with outbreaks:

- If you have a cold sore, you should
- Do replace your toothbrush with a fresh one.
- When you're under a lot of stress, get plenty of rest, vitamin C, and zinc tablets.
- To protect your skin from the sun, wind, and cold, use a hypoallergenic, clear lip balm.

- Do not share or drink your cup or drink during the emergency.
- Do not attempt to pop, drain, or otherwise interfere with the healing of a cold sore.

If you have genital herpes, follow these steps:

- Wear cotton underwear and loose-fitting clothes.
- Do take long, hot showers and keep the surrounding area clean and dry at all times.
- Do not take a bath or relax in a hot tub.

I haven't had sex in a long time. Even if you use a condom, the virus might be transmitted.

# CHAPTER 4

## Foods to Avoid When You Have a Cold Sore

Cold sores can be excruciatingly painful and cause social embarrassment. While the blisters around your mouth may prohibit you from eating your normal meals, there are some foods that cause no discomfort but help prolong the outbreak's duration.

### *Food that is acidic*

Eating acidic foods might worsen cold sores that scab and resurface. Citrus fruits, tomatoes, fruit juices, alcohol, soda, pickles, and vinegar-based salad dressings are all foods to avoid. Hot and spicy foods have a proclivity for breaking cold sores. We advise consuming warm foods and limiting salt and spice intake.

### *Food that has been processed*

During a cold sore breakout, certain foods decrease your immune system. A cold sore may recur as a result of this. Sugary breakfast cereals, packaged snacks, frozen foods, canned foods, pasta meals, and high-calorie snacks should all be avoided.

### Foods high in arginine

Cold sores are caused by the herpes simplex virus, which requires arginine (an amino acid) to proliferate and thrive in your body. Depriving a virus of arginine will very likely cut the length and severity of an outbreak. Flaxseeds, sunflower seeds, sesame seeds, chocolate, spinach, whole grains, almonds, peanuts, hazelnuts, and walnuts are all high in arginine. When you first notice the signs of a cold sore, stay away from these foods totally.

### What am I allowed to eat?

Once you have a cold sore outbreak, there is no way to stop it. You can eat foods that aid in the prevention of breakouts. The amino acid lysine binds to arginine and prevents the virus from reproducing. Vegetables, beans, milk, cheese, and fish are high in lysine, which helps to improve your immune system and prevent cold sores.

Cold foods, vegetable juices, and warm soups can satisfy your hunger while keeping the sore from becoming worse during an epidemic.

# CHAPTER 5

## How do I obtain herpes treatment?

Despite the fact that there is no cure for herpes, there are a variety of treatments available to alleviate the symptoms and control the infection. Herpes treatment speeds up the healing process and/or reduces the frequency with which outbreaks recur. Your doctor will advise you on the best treatment options for your specific circumstances. If you're having an outbreak, your doctor may be able to prescribe medication to help your sores heal faster. You can also help to alleviate the discomfort by:

- Soak in a hot tub
- Maintaining a dry genital area (moisture makes the sores last longer)
- Put on loose, comfortable clothing.
- putting an ice pack on the sores

- Use aspirin, ibuprofen (Advil, Motrin), or acetaminophen as a pain reliever (Tylenol).

**What can I do to avoid herpes outbreaks?**

If you have a lot of herpes outbreaks, your doctor may recommend suppressive therapy, which involves taking medicine every day. It can help you avoid having herpes outbreaks in the future and make it less likely that your friends will get them, too. Taking care of yourself by eating good foods, getting enough sleep, and avoiding stress, whether or not you use drugs to treat herpes, may help prevent recurrent outbreaks.

Nobody knows for sure what causes outbreaks of genital herpes. Outbreaks can be caused by other illnesses, surgery, sex, your period, skin irritations, and stress. Flare-ups of oral herpes can be caused by sunburns, lip injuries, or other illnesses. If you have oral herpes, try to avoid becoming sunburned.

Genital herpes episodes tend to happen less often and get

shorter and weaker as time goes on, even if you don't get treated.

**What happens if you don't seek treatment for herpes?**
The good news is that herpes isn't fatal or even extremely harmful. Herpes is painful, but unlike other STDs, it doesn't get worse over time or cause major health issues.

If you don't get treated for herpes, you may continue to have outbreaks on a regular basis, or they may only occur infrequently. After a while, some people stop experiencing outbreaks on their own.

People may choose not to seek treatment for a variety of reasons. They may not experience as many breakouts as others, or their outbreaks may not affect them as much. Or perhaps they aren't having sex right now and aren't concerned about contracting herpes. Treatment for herpes can be obtained regardless of your circumstances.

Because the sores provide HIV with an open conduit into your body, having herpes can make it simpler to contract

HIV. Always wear condoms to help prevent the spread of both herpes and HIV.

## *How to Stay Away From Herpes*

Sexual skin-to-skin contact with someone who has genital herpes, including vaginal, anal, and oral sex, is how it spreads. As a result, the best strategy to avoid contracting herpes and other STDs is to avoid coming into contact with another person's mouth or genitals.

However, because almost everyone has sex at some point in their lives, learning how to have safer sex is essential. When having sex, you should use condoms and dental dams to protect yourself from getting an STD.

Condoms won't always protect you against herpes because they can live on parts of your body that aren't protected by them (including the scrotum, butt cheeks, upper thighs, and labia). They do, however, reduce your chances of contracting herpes.

During an outbreak of herpes, avoid having sex with

anyone because that's when it's easiest to spread. Herpes can spread even if there are no sores or symptoms, so use condoms and dental dams even if everything appears to be in order.

## *How can I ensure that I don't infect anyone with herpes?*

Try not to be alarmed if you discover you have herpes. In a few ways, you can prevent HPV from spreading to your partners and other parts of your body. During oral, anal, and vaginal sex, always use condoms and dental dams. Consult your doctor about taking herpes medication on a daily basis to reduce your risk of spreading the virus.

Even if you're using a condom, don't have sex during a herpes outbreak. There could be sores where the condom doesn't reach.

Learn how to spot an outbreak coming on and quit having sex as soon as you detect the warning signals. You might feel a burning, itchy, or tingling sensation that means you're going to get a sore. Wait until your sores are completely healed and the scabs have fallen off before having sex. Because you can spread the illness to other regions of your body or other people if you touch your herpes sores, don't touch them. If you touch a sore, immediately wash your hands with soap and water.

Contact lenses can become wet if you spit on them. This could spread oral herpes to your eyes. Don't kiss anyone if you have a cold sore in your mouth, especially babies, children, or pregnant women.

Before you have sex, always tell your sexual partners that you have herpes so that you can work together to keep it from spreading. It's difficult to tell someone you have an STD, although herpes is extremely common and does not cause major health problems. As a result, try not to be overly humiliated or upset about it.

Patients with herpes are twice as likely to contract HIV as those who do not. People who have both herpes and HIV are far more likely to spread the virus to their partners. As a result, it's critical to use condoms to protect yourself and your partner.

**What should I do if I'm diagnosed with herpes?**

It's natural to experience a range of emotions after learning that you have herpes. At first, you may feel angry, embarrassed, ashamed, or upset. But as time passes, you'll probably feel a lot better and realize that having herpes isn't such a huge problem. Herpes patients have relationships and lead completely normal lives. Herpes can be treated, and there's a lot you can do to ensure that you don't pass it on to anyone you have sex with.

Herpes affects millions of individuals worldwide, so you're not alone. The majority of people contract at least one STD over their lives and having herpes or any STD is nothing to be ashamed of. It doesn't make you "dirty" or a nasty person; it just implies that you're a regular person who contracted a rather common infection. Herpes may strike anyone who has ever been kissed on the lips or had sex—and that includes a lot of people.

Herpes is not fatal, and it seldom causes major health concerns. Herpes outbreaks are inconvenient and unpleasant, but the first one is usually the worst. For many people, outbreaks become less frequent over time and may eventually cease. Even if the virus remains in your body for the rest of your life, that doesn't mean you'll always have sores. When you find out you have herpes, the best thing you can do is follow your doctor's treatment recommendations. If you're having trouble dealing with the news, talking to a close friend or joining a herpes support group may help you feel better.

Also, inform anyone with whom you have intercourse that you have herpes. It's not the easiest conversation to have, but it's crucial.

### *What should I say to people when they find out I have herpes?*

It may be frightening to acknowledge you have herpes, but talking about it can help you feel better. You could confide in a close friend who is nonjudgmental and trustworthy to keep the conversation confidential. Other family members, such as parents, brothers and sisters, aunts, uncles, and cousins, can also be a source of consolation. Herpes is really common, so it's probable that the person you're speaking with has it as well.

There are a lot of online support groups for people who have herpes, and the American Sexual Health Association has a list of support groups in your area.

### *What should I know about dating while having herpes?*

When people learn they have herpes, they may believe their love lives are finished, but this is simply not the case. Herpes patients have romantic and sexual relationships with one another or with non-herpes partners.

Talking about STDs isn't the most enjoyable topic to discuss. However, it's important to always tell your partners if you have herpes so that you can help stop the disease from spreading.

There is no one-size-fits-all approach to discussing an STD, but here are some suggestions:

- *Maintain your composure and carry on.* Herpes affects millions of people, many of whom are in partnership. Herpes isn't a big concern for most couples. Try to have a calm and optimistic demeanor throughout the chat. Herpes is merely a medical condition; it says nothing about you as a person.
- *Make it a two-way dialogue.* Keep in mind that STDs are extremely frequent, so who knows? It's possible that your partner has herpes as well. Begin by asking if they've ever been tested for an STD or if they've ever had one.
- *You know what you're talking about.* There is a lot of misinformation about herpes out there, so educate yourself and be ready to correct the record. Let your partner know that there are treatments for

herpes and measures to prevent it from spreading during sex.

- ***Consider the timing.*** Choose a time when you won't be distracted or interrupted, as well as a private and relaxing location. If you're scared, talk it over with a friend or practice speaking in front of a mirror. Speaking the words out loud may seem foolish, but it might help you know what you want to say and feel more secure while speaking with your spouse.

First and foremost, put your safety first. Telling a partner you're worried they'll hurt you in person might not be safe. You're probably better off sending them an e-mail, text message, or calling them—or, in the worst-case scenario, not telling them at all. If you believe you are in danger, call 1-800-799-SAFE or go to the National Domestic Violence Hotline website for assistance.

So, when do you reveal your herpes status to your new crush? You don't have to tell them the first time you hang out with them, but you should inform them before you have sex with them. So when you feel like you can trust the person and the relationship is headed in that direction, it's definitely a good moment.

It's natural to be concerned about your partner's reaction. There's no getting around it: some folks are going to flip out. If this occurs, be cool and discuss all of the options for preventing the spread of herpes. It's understandable if you need to give your partner some time and space to process the news. And most people are aware that herpes is extremely prevalent but not a serious illness.

When speaking with your partner, try not to play the blame game. It's not always a sign that someone cheated if one of you gets herpes for the first time throughout the relationship. Herpes symptoms might appear days, weeks, months, or even years after you've contracted the virus. As a result, determining when and where someone contracted herpes is often difficult. The most important thing is that both of you are put to the test. If it turns out that only one of you has herpes, talk about how to keep it from spreading. Also, inform your previous partners so that they can be checked.

***Will my pregnancy be affected if I have herpes?***

If you've had genital herpes for a long time and become pregnant, don't be concerned; it's rare that you'll pass herpes on to your baby during delivery. If you're pregnant, though, you should always tell your doctor if you have genital herpes.

It's much more harmful to obtain herpes when pregnant, especially late in the pregnancy. It may result in a miscarriage or an early delivery. If you infect your baby with herpes while he or she is still in the womb, it can result in brain damage or vision difficulties. If you have herpes sores when you go into labor, your doctor may recommend a C-section to prevent the virus from infecting your baby during delivery.

If your partner has herpes but you don't, avoid

unprotected vaginal, anal, or oral intercourse while pregnant, as this is the most common way to contract the disease. Your doctor may advise your partner to take herpes medication while you're pregnant so they don't pass the virus on to you. To discover more about how to avoid acquiring herpes, read "How to Prevent Herpes."

During pregnancy or childbirth, oral herpes is not harmful. If you have a cold sore after giving birth, however, wait until the sore has completely healed before kissing your baby.

## *How do you keep herpes from spreading in your sexual relationships?*

If you have genital herpes, there are certain things you can do on your own to protect your spouse from infection. The most important considerations are:

- During an epidemic, don't have sex, use condoms when you don't have symptoms, and talk about the disease openly with your partner.

- People who frequently have genital herpes may benefit from antiviral treatment as a preventive measure. This drug reduces the danger of infecting others by inhibiting the virus's activity.

## Herpes symptoms and signs

Herpes causes painful skin sores in both types of people. Herpes symptoms include:

- *Sores in the mouth caused by the herpes virus:* HSV-1, often known as cold sores, causes painful sores that resemble blisters at first. They finally rupture and form a crust on the surface. The sores normally cure within a week to ten days.
- *Sores caused by genital herpes:* The lesions in the vaginal area might be caused by HSV-1 or HSV-2. They begin as painful blisters, then dry up and heal over time, much like mouth sores.

### Other Ailments

Herpes sores can form anywhere on the body, though

they frequently appear around the mouth or genitals.

## *Symptoms of the flu*

Other symptoms, like fever, fatigue, and body aches, may also happen during a herpes outbreak. Not everyone with herpes has recurrent outbreaks. Some people may have a single outbreak and then show no symptoms for the rest of their lives. It's possible that the virus will remain dormant in their bodies.

## *Causes of the Herpes Virus*

Both types of herpes can be contracted through direct contact with an infected person. Even if they don't have symptoms, HSV-1 carriers can pass it on through direct contact. The virus can be spread by skin-to-skin contact. By touching an open herpes sore and then touching another portion of your skin, herpes can be spread to other regions, including your eyes. Avoid touching sores and wash your hands as soon as possible if you do.

## *Having sexual contact*

Sexual interaction is the most common way for people to

contract HSV-2. Herpes can be transmitted through oral, anal, and genital intercourse. Even if your partner has no symptoms of HSV-2, you can contract it. HSV-1 can also be transmitted to your genitals during oral sex.

## *Pregnancy*

Herpes can be passed down to offspring by pregnant moms. This can lead to major issues in some circumstances. If you're expecting a child, talk to your doctor about your herpes risk.

Many people contract HSV-1 as babies or children through non-sexual contact with the virus-infected saliva of an adult. Herpes can affect anyone, although people with compromised immune systems are more likely to contract it. Periodic outbreaks occur in some people. These eruptions can be triggered by other ailments like sun exposure, menstrual periods, or stress. Most people discover that their first breakout is the most severe. The virus transfers from skin cells to nerve cells during that outbreak, where it will remain indefinitely. Later outbreaks are less severe and painful. Some people experience a tingling feeling before a fresh outbreak begins.

## *What are the symptoms of genital herpes?*

The genital herpes virus is transmitted through saliva, sperm, and vaginal fluids. It is possible to contract genital herpes from someone who is asymptomatic. You could have the infection and be unaware of it, infecting someone else. Herpes genitalis can be spread by:

- Anal, vaginal-penile, and vaginal-vaginal intercourse are all examples of intercourse.
- Oral intercourse (providing or receiving) with an infected person.
- ejaculation-free skin-to-skin contact.
- Touching raw sores, including when breastfeeding, is not a good idea.
- A mother or gestational parent with an active infection gives birth to a child.

- Objects such as toilet seats cannot transmit genital herpes.

However, genital herpes can be transmitted through shared sex toys. To be safe, always wash sex toys before and after use and never share them. If you do, use a condom to keep them safe.

**What causes genital herpes to appear?**

Symptoms are frequently at their worst during the first outbreak or flare-up (called primary herpes). Symptoms usually develop two to twenty days following the infection. Symptoms can continue for up to four weeks if they are active. You might have the following symptoms:

- Fever, chills, lethargy, and body aches are flu-like symptoms.
- Itching, burning, or irritation in the genital area.
- Blisters or sores in the vaginal area that are painful and break open.
- Headaches
- It's urination that hurts (dysuria).

- lymph nodes that are swollen.

# CHAPTER 6

## What causes female vaginal sores?

Female genital sores can be caused by a variety of factors. Sexually transmitted infections (STIs), such as herpes, are the most frequent. STI-related genital sores are often painful and irritating. They might appear as a single sore or a cluster of sores. These are the most common genital sores, and they are extremely contagious. Some vulva and vaginal pimples are innocuous, while others are itchy, unpleasant, or uncomfortable. Some of them may emit a discharge. It might be difficult to distinguish between STIs that cause vaginal sores and those that do not. As a result, anyone suffering from genital sores should seek medical attention for a proper diagnosis and treatment.

Genital herpes is a sexually transmitted infection (STI) that creates sores on the genitals. This prevalent virus affects more than 1 in 6 people aged 14 to 49 in the

United States. It is one of the most common causes of vaginal sores. During a genital herpes outbreak, one or more tiny blister-like lesions will appear around the genitals or rectum. Blisters break open, resulting in painful genital sores. It normally takes a week or more for the sores to heal. Because most people with genital herpes have no or minor symptoms, they are unaware that they have it. This makes it simple to pass from one person to the next. Although genital herpes is not curable, the number of outbreaks tends to decrease over time. Medications can help people shorten outbreaks, and some treatments can cut the risk of passing the virus on to sexual partners by a lot.

### *Syphilis*

Syphilis is a sexually transmitted infection (STI) that causes one or more painless ulcers known as chancres. They're usually spherical and firm. Treponema pallidum is the organism that causes syphilis. Chancres usually emerge 10–90 days following bacterial contact. The ulcers usually go away in 3–6 weeks. Syphilis, on the other hand, can have catastrophic consequences if left untreated. Syphilis can be treated with an intravenous course of penicillin G. A person may need to have another test after therapy to ensure that the infection has gone away.

## *Chancroid*

Chancroid is a sexually transmitted infection (STI) that causes painful genital sores and enlarged lymph glands in the groin area. Haemophilus ducreyi is the bacteria that causes it. Chancroid lesions begin as little red bumps that swiftly expand into pustules or pus-filled pimples. These pustules explode, resulting in excruciatingly painful sores. Ulcers have a tendency to bleed freely. If left untreated, ulcers can linger for 1–3 months. It takes 4–10 days for chancroid to appear following sexual interaction, but it might take up to 35 days.

Symptoms normally improve within three days of starting medication, and the infection clears up within seven days. Large ulcers might take up to two weeks to heal.

## *Contagiosum Molluscum*

Contagious: Molluscum contagiosum is a skin infection that affects the lower parts of the body. It causes small sores or lumps.

The lesions can also arise on the genitals and around the anus, and they can grow into larger, itchy, and tender sores. They come in a variety of colors, including flesh, gray-white, yellow, and pink. The lesions might last anywhere from two weeks to four years.

The majority of lesions cure on their own, while some may reappear. They can be removed by doctors so that they don't spread to other people.

## *Inguinal Granuloma*

Granuloma inguinale is a sexually transmitted infection (STI) that creates bleedy, deep red sores. These ulcers, on the other hand, are usually painless. Klebsiella granulomatis is the organism that causes the infection.

Granuloma inguinale is uncommon in the United States. Antibiotics can be used to treat this infection, but it may return 6–18 months later.

## Causes other than STIs

Although STIs are the most common cause of genital sores, there are a few other possibilities. When genital sores are very rare, they could be cancerous cysts that can be removed by a doctor. Other causes of female genital sores that aren't caused by STIs include:

- Genital ulcers that aren't caused by sexual activity
- NSAGU (non-sexually acquired genital ulceration) is a disorder in which painful ulcers form around the genitals. Females are more likely than males to have recurrent instances.

Ulcers can appear as a single shallow round sore or as a cluster of shallow round sores. They can show up in women often or not at all. They can show up on a regular basis, like before menstruation each month.

The specific cause of NSAGU is unknown, but it appears

to be linked to immune system function and underlying medical problems such as celiac disease or Crohn's disease.

## Hidradenitis suppurativa is a type of suppurative hydradenitis.

Hidradenitis suppurativa is a persistent skin disorder characterized by pus-filled pimples, hard lumps, or open sores that do not drain. These lumps and sores can form on the surface of the skin as well as beneath it.

The bumps usually appear in places where the skin scrapes against itself, such as the groin and armpits. They can be quite large and extremely painful.

### *Psoriasis*

Psoriasis is an excess of skin cells that causes a persistent skin disorder. Psoriasis comes in a variety of forms, some of which might result in skin sores. For example, pustular psoriasis causes white, pus-filled blisters that might break and turn into open sores. The skin may become scaly after the blisters have disappeared. On the other hand, guttate psoriasis is characterized by little dot-like lesions that spread throughout the skin.

Behcet's disease is a condition that affects people. Behcet's illness is a rare inflammatory disease that causes ulcers in the mouth and genitals, skin lesions, and vision problems in people.

Ulcers are often round or oval, with reddish edges. They usually affect the vulva in females. They normally heal in a few days, although they might pop up and disappear at any time. The exact cause of Behcet's disease is unknown, but it is thought to be linked to heredity.

# CHAPTER 7

## How do you deal with herpes on a long-term basis?

If you have a lot of outbreaks in a year, you might want to think about suppression treatment. Antiviral lotions for cold sores are available in pharmacies, but if the sore lasts longer than 5-7 days, you should consult a doctor.

Your doctor may send you to a sexual health clinic for genital herpes treatment.

An acute, short-term infection is easily treated by taking antiviral medications over a period of time. Antiviral pills come in a variety of shapes and sizes. Some courses are more intense and only require 1 to 2 days of study, while others require 5 days. If you develop new symptoms during treatment or if your treatment does not entirely heal your symptoms, you may require additional treatment. If this occurs, you should consult your doctor.

Oral herpes (cold sores) management:

Refrain from making direct physical contact with others. Cups, silverware, make-up, and lip balm are among the items that might spread the infection. Communal facilities such as showers, toilets, and swimming pools are still available.

**Neither oral sex nor kissing are acceptable.**

After applying antiviral cream or contacting the sore, wash your hands well with soap and water; avoid touching the sore unless you need to apply medication.

Managing genital herpes—avoid having sex during a genital herpes outbreak or during the early stages of an outbreak (when you start getting symptoms of genital herpes). Precautions like these will help to keep it from spreading to other people:

- If you've been diagnosed with herpes but don't have any symptoms, use a condom because the virus can still be transmitted to your partner through direct skin contact even if you're wearing one.

- Allow no one to come into direct contact with your blisters or sores.
- If you use sex toys, make sure they're clean and covered with a condom.

Notifying a partner that you have herpes:

- Many people are unaware of what herpes is and how widespread it is. It is critical for partners to be honest with one another in order to discuss these issues openly. Many people will appreciate and support honesty.
- Your unique style will influence what you say. When it comes to bringing up the subject, there are good times and bad ones. It's not a good idea to bring it up right before intercourse.
- If you think you'll have sex on your first date, it's a good idea to bring it up during your date. Otherwise, you might want to wait a while for trust

and comfort to grow between the two of you before deciding to discuss it.
- Choose a time when you are feeling good about yourself and have a positive outlook on life. This will give you and your partner time to talk about it honestly.

You can make some lifestyle adjustments to help lower the risk of breakouts, but many triggers in everyday life are inevitable. The following are some examples of probable triggers:

Stress is a common trigger that can manifest as both emotional and physical stress (for example, during surgery). Excessive stress can wreak havoc on your immune system, triggering both oral and genital herpes.

*Weak immune system:* If you have a compromised immune system, you are more susceptible to outbreaks. People who have HIV, cancer, or diabetes are at a higher risk.

During intercourse, vaginal friction might cause an

outbreak. If this bothers you, make sure you use enough lubricant during intercourse.

*Fever:-* When you have a fever, your body is put under physical strain. When you have a fever, you're more likely to have oral herpes, which can cause "fever blisters" around your mouth.

Tight clothing should be avoided because it might cause vaginal irritation, which can lead to an outbreak.

*Hormones:* Due to fluctuations in hormone levels, some women report having more frequent outbreaks before or after their periods.

*Sunlight or sunbed use:* it is unknown how sunlight causes an outbreak, but if you are sensitive, wear appropriate sunscreen whenever you are exposed to the sun. Oral herpes is the most common type of herpes.

*Avoiding triggers:-* if you notice a pattern of triggers, make changes to your lifestyle or limit your exposure to them.

Excessive use of the amino acid arginine might cause an

epidemic. Avoid arginine-rich foods like almonds and chocolate. A diet high in the amino acid lysine has also been shown to help prevent outbreaks and stop the herpes virus from multiplying. The following are some examples of lysine-rich foods that can help:

- Dairy products, especially yogurt and cheese,
- Meat and fish, especially high-protein meats like chicken and beef,
- Apples, apricots, and pears, in particular,
- Beans and cruciferous vegetables, such as broccoli, are examples of vegetables.

impact on the emotions:

A cold sore in your mouth can be very painful, and genital herpes can have a big effect on your life and relationships, so you need to be careful.

Most people adjust to living with herpes after some time. At first, you may have feelings of humiliation, rage, or anxiety, but it's critical to give yourself time to adjust.

If you're frightened, anxious, or sad about your diagnosis,

talk to your doctor. They may advise you to seek counseling or additional assistance.

# CHAPTER 8

## At-home herpes treatment

Herpes is a viral-borne infection caused by the herpes simplex virus. There is no cure for this at this time, but there are many therapies, such as home remedies, that can help ease the symptoms.

Sores on the skin are a symptom of herpes. Typically, the illness affects the mouth, genitals, and anal areas.

Herpes simplex virus 1 (HSV-1) and herpes simplex virus 2 (HSV-2) are the two forms of herpes simplex virus (HSV-2). HSV-1 and HSV-2 are both capable of causing genital herpes. According to a reliable source, only HSV-1 causes oral herpes. A source you can trust.

This guide outlines many home remedies that may aid in the management of herpes symptoms, as well as some shopping possibilities. It will also go through how to avoid getting sick and when to see a doctor.

## Compresses

A hot or cold compress can help with the irritation and agony of a herpes lesion. To keep blisters from forming during an oral herpes infection, apply heat to the area around the lips and the inside of the mouth, too,

It's simple to make a cold compress at home. Wrap an ice pack in a flannel and place it on the hurting spot.

Do not, however, place the ice pack directly on the skin. It's also a good idea to gently cleanse the region with saltwater.

Cool compresses can also help people who have eye herpes, according to the American Academy of Ophthalmology. They can help people with eye herpes reduce pain, irritation, and swelling in the eyelid area.

### *Honey*

According to a 2019 study, kanuka honey may be just as efficient as antiviral lotions in treating oral herpes.

In the research, antiviral cream took 8 days to heal the

lesions, while honey took 9 days. Oral herpes can improve without therapy in 1–2 weeks, and the study did not include a control group.

It's also uncertain whether the possible healing capabilities of kanuka honey are unique to it or if they'd be present in any honey.

### Where can I get it?

Kanuka honey can be purchased from a variety of companies online. Here's an example:

- Kanuka Honey from Tahi
- The white blossoms of the kanuka tree in New Zealand are used to make this raw kanuka honey.

According to the company, raw honey is 100 percent natural, unpasteurized, and free of added water, sugar, chemicals, or preservatives.

Tahi further claims that it produces this honey in an ethical and sustainable manner. The honey is carbon-negative and biodiversity-positive, and the company's headquarters are powered entirely by solar energy.

All of the proceeds from the sale of this honey go to environmental, community, and cultural causes.

### *Garlic*

Viruses, including both types of HSV, can be slowed down by garlic, according to Trusted Source.

According to Trusted Source, allicin, a chemical found in garlic, maybe beneficial against HSV. Garlic, on the other hand, has no clear proof that it can prevent, cure, or treat herpes.

While garlic may have antiviral benefits, research shows that it also contains volatile organic sulfur compounds. When raw garlic is applied to the skin, these chemicals can cause burns. Leg burns are prevalent, according to the Dr Sebi.

When using raw garlic topically on the skin and surrounding mucous membranes like the eyes, mouth, and nose, people should be cautious of the danger of burns. If a person's skin becomes irritated, they should stop using it right away and thoroughly wash the affected area. Garlic can be used in many ways, such as eating raw garlic and taking garlic capsules.

### *Where can I get it?*

Garlic capsules and pills are available for purchase online from a variety of companies. As an example, consider the following:

- Garlic 2000 mg from Nature's Bounty
- These tablets have an enteric coating and are odorless. The manufacturer says that the enteric coating keeps the tablets together until they reach the small intestine.

According to Nature's Bounty, each pill includes 400 milligrams (mg) of garlic extract, which is equivalent to 2000 milligrams (mg) of raw garlic, according to Nature's Bounty. People should take one pill up to three times per day with food, according to the manufacturer.

## *Vitamins*

There are several vitamins that may help protect the body from the virus and help with the symptoms, too. If a person's vitamin D levels are low, herpes infections are more likely to recur. Vitamin D improves the part of the immune system, which helps to protect the body from infection. If you take Vitamin E, it may help your body fight off illnesses like herpes, which can make you more vulnerable to infection. Vitamin E, is currently being tested in clinical trials to treat herpes.

There is also continuing study into vitamin C's antiviral capabilities. According to retrospective research, oral vitamin C in combination with antiviral medication may minimize the recurrence of herpes simplex keratitis, a corneal infection caused by HSV.

### *Where can I get it?*

The following companies and websites sell vitamin supplements:

- D3 (Vegan) Liquid by Pure Encapsulations

- This vitamin D3 tincture is gluten-free and has no GMOs, making it safe for vegetarians and vegans

This product, according to Pure Encapsulations, may assist in improving cardiovascular and immunological health, as well as supporting bone, prostate, and colon function. This tincture comes in a 5 drop serving quantity. Vitamin D3 is present in each serving in the amount of 25 micrograms (mcg).

## Garden of Life Vitamin Code Raw

### *Vitamin E 60 capsules*

GMOs, synthetic binders, fillers, or artificial flavors are not present in these raw vitamin E capsules. Fat-soluble vitamins A, D, K, and selenium are also included in this formulation. These vitamin supplements, according to Garden of Life, can assist in promoting ocular and immunological health. People should take two capsules daily, with or without food, according to the manufacturer. Breaking the capsules open and adding the powder to liquids is also an option. The following is the nutritional information for each serving size:

- 900 micrograms of vitamin A.
- 50 micrograms of vitamin D.
- Vitamin E (125 mg)
- 72 micrograms of vitamin K
- 61 micrograms of selenium

## *Nordic Naturals Vitamin C gummies*

These vitamin C gummies are recommended for those aged 4 and up. The gummies are GMO-free, vegetarian, and vegan. According to Nordic Naturals, these candies may have antioxidant characteristics that can help boost a person's immune system. According to the business, people should take two gummies a day with food. Vitamin C is present in each gummy in the amount of 250 mg. Nordic Naturals Vitamin C Gummies were $13.45 at the time of publication. The company also offers a subscription service to help customers save money on their purchases.

## *Gels*

Applying petroleum jelly to the affected area of genital herpes can help relieve the pain of peeing. Before and after applying the jelly, make sure to wash your hands. For herpes outbreaks, doctors may also prescribe prescription gels or ointments.

### *Where can I get it?*

Vaseline is a well-known brand of petroleum jelly that can be found in many stores and online.

- Vaseline is a 100 percent pure petroleum jelly.
- Vaseline is available for purchase on Amazon.

This 13-ounce product is hypoallergenic and suitable for sensitive and dry skin. According to Vaseline, the cream helps seal in moisture, which may aid in natural skin healing. Petroleum jelly also serves as a barrier between the skin and the elements.

## *Dietary Modifications*

Pomegranate has been used as a home treatment for infection for generations. Zinc in pomegranates can aid in the reduction of herpes infections. Pomegranates also have antibacterial, anti-inflammatory, and antioxidant activities. These characteristics may help the immune system. The following are some other dietary suggestions:

- Increasing lysine intake, while data for its usefulness is conflicting.
- Avoid arginine as an amino acid.
- Avoid excessive smoking, red wine, and caffeine consumption.
- Food allergens must be identified and eliminated.
- Soy protein, peanuts, walnuts, and salmon are all excellent providers of this nutrient.
- Arginine from a reliable source lysine can be found in avocados, poultry, cottage cheese, and pork.

## Supplements

According to Trusted Source, the following supplements may help manage herpes symptoms:

- Lysine
- Zinc
- Adenosine monophosphate
- Lemon balm is an herb that has been used for centuries.
- Vitamin C
- A source of vitamin e.

Experts discovered in a 2017 review that taking a minimum of 1 gram of lysine per day, combined with a low-arginine diet, can help patients control their symptoms. Before taking any supplements, consult your doctor. They may have negative side effects or interact with other drugs. Because the Food and Drug Administration (FDA) does not regulate supplements, it's not always easy to know exactly what's in them.

### *Where can I get it?*

Lysine supplements are available from the following companies:

- At CVS Pharmacy, 1000 mg L-Lysine caplets

There is no yeast, wheat, or gluten in these vegetarian caplets. They also don't have milk or lactose in them, as well as other allergies. According to CVS Pharmacy, these caplets may assist in healthy skin, collagen formation, and tissue maintenance. On an empty stomach, the business recommends taking one caplet each day. L-lysine is 1000 milligrams in each caplet.

### *Thorne Zinc Picolinate 30 mg*

These capsules are gluten-free, dairy-free, and soy-free. According to Thorne, these supplements may help with immune health, reproductive health, and more. One capsule per day is recommended by the manufacturer. Zinc is present in each capsule in the amount of 30 milligrams.

### *Oils*

Certain essential oils have been shown to decrease viral spread in HSV-1 cells. Oils that may be beneficial include:

- Thyme in the garden
- Zataria multiflora is a flowering plant.
- Eucalyptus caesia is a kind of eucalyptus.
- rosemary
- Wormwood
- Cypress hinoki
- Tripterygium hypoglaucum is a medicinal herb.

Components found in clove oil, cinnamon essential oil, and basil essential oil. Oils can be diffused, diluted in a carrier oil, added to a bath, or massaged directly into the skin. Essential oils should not be consumed because some are poisonous and can cause harm. When utilizing aromatherapy, keep in mind anyone else in the vicinity. Some essential oils are toxic to pets and women who are pregnant or nursing. It's crucial to use a carrier oil because using essential oils directly on the skin can have negative consequences. Almond oil and olive oil are examples of carrier oils. Researchers are also testing other home remedies, like sesame oil, organic coconut oil, and jojoba oil, to see if they can help. There isn't enough research to say whether or not a certain oil can assist someone in managing herpes symptoms.

### *Medication*

Some drugs can help prevent the herpes virus from spreading and reduce the severity and frequency of symptoms. Antiviral medications are the most common treatments prescribed by doctors for this purpose. Acyclovir, famciclovir, valacyclovir, and penciclovir are among them. Acyclovir can help people with genital herpes have fewer first-time or recurring outbreaks. It also helps people with chickenpox and shingles heal faster by reducing discomfort and speeding up the healing process. Acyclovir and valacyclovir are two antiviral drugs that require less frequent administration than acyclovir. These drugs, however, are not licensed for use in children. Antiviral drugs can be taken by mouth, injected, or applied to the skin by a doctor.

In rare circumstances, a doctor may recommend oral medication over topical treatment. For example, oral acyclovir, valacyclovir, and famciclovir are more successful than topical versions of the drugs in treating herpes labialis, according to a 2017 study.

**Telehealth companies that operate online**

Herpes medicines are available online from the following companies:

- Blink Health is a company that specializes in providing health care.
- Telemedicine service: Acyclovir, valacyclovir, and famciclovir are some of the prescription herpes medicines that can be bought through this service.

To use this service, people must have a current prescription or contact a doctor online through Blink Health. Blink Health provides home delivery, or medication can be picked up at a local drugstore. Walmart Pharmacy, Safeway, and Albertson's are just a few of the 35,000 pharmacies that the corporation works with.

### *Lemonaid*

This telemedicine company sells herpes drugs on prescription. People will be required to complete an online health questionnaire and show photo identification. This will set you back $25. Lemonaid may require a video or telephone consultation with a healthcare expert, depending on the state in which a person lives.

The organization offers a one-year prescription for prophylactic treatment as well as urgent treatment for breakouts. People can have their medications delivered to their homes or picked up at a nearby drugstore.

### **Prevention**

Herpes causes no symptoms in the majority of instances. However, if a person has any symptoms, it is best not to have oral, anal, or vaginal sex. A condom is a little piece of plastic that is used. It may not be enough to stop transmission completely.

It's advisable to have an open conversation about herpes with a new sexual partner and to think about getting tested. If one person has been diagnosed with herpes, they should tell all of their recent sexual partners, because they may need to be tested and treated as well.

### *When should you see a doctor?*

If a person has had sex with someone who has herpes or if they have any symptoms, they should contact a doctor for testing. If a person with herpes becomes pregnant, they should seek medical advice. Although uncommon, the herpes virus can infect a fetus before, during, or shortly after delivery. This could result in newborn herpes, which is potentially fatal.

# Acknowledgments

The Glory of this book's success goes to God Almighty and my beautiful Family, Fans, Readers & well-wishers, Customers, and Friends for their endless support and encouragement.

Printed in the USA
CPSIA information can be obtained
at www.ICGtesting.com
LVHW040059090124
768362LV00010B/661

9 781685 220594